YOUR KNOWLEDGE HAS VALUE

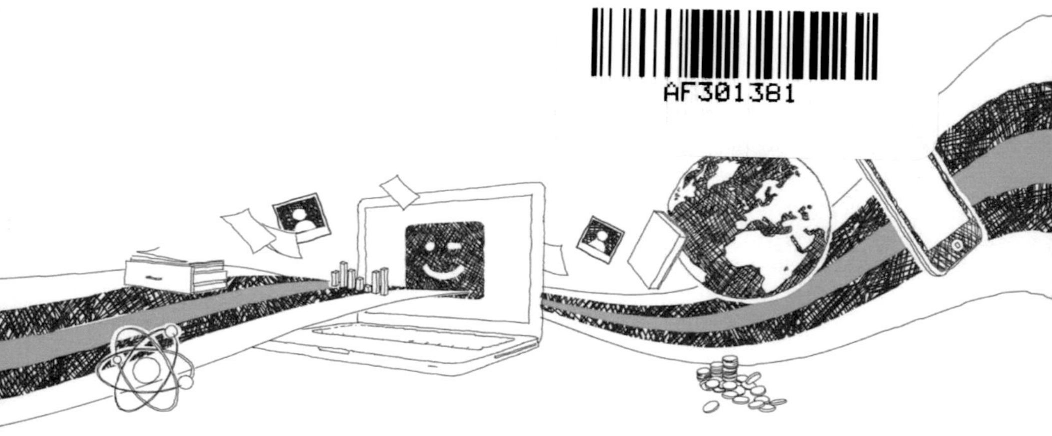

- We will publish your bachelor's and
  master's thesis, essays and papers

- Your own eBook and book -
  sold worldwide in all relevant shops

- Earn money with each sale

Upload your text at www.GRIN.com
and publish for free

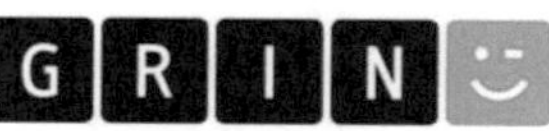

Bibliographic information published by the German National Library:

The German National Library lists this publication in the National Bibliography; detailed bibliographic data are available on the Internet at http://dnb.dnb.de .

Imprint:

Copyright © 2015 GRIN Verlag, Open Publishing GmbH
Print and binding: Books on Demand GmbH, Norderstedt Germany
ISBN: 9783668277427

This book at GRIN:

http://www.grin.com/en/e-book/338007/aromatherapy-as-stress-relief

Denny Kyaloh

Aromatherapy as stress relief

GRIN Publishing

Use of Aromatherapy in Stress Reduction

Abstract

The use of traditional medicine has not always been the only means to deliver healing and treatment. Many other methods and forms of medication have been used in various parts of the world for a long time. With the complexity of ailments and increase of the number of patients, doctors are now exploring the alternative forms of medication. One of these methods is aromatherapy. This form of alternative medicine is being embraced to deliver treatment to those that are heavily laden with stress and depression. This paper takes a deep look at the various forms of research that have been published on the effectiveness of the treatment. Through the examination of the various literatures published by experts in the field, the paper shows why aromatherapy is becoming a widely accepted form of alternative medicine. The paper also explores the causes of stress and why stress is such a serious problem that needs the radical intervention of medical experts.

Contents

Introduction

Aromatherapy is the use of aromatic plant oils in various healing processes including mood boosting and stress relieving. Aromatic plants are also referred to as fragrant or essential oils. The processing of the oils is done in such as way that the oils are highly concentrated to make sure that just a few drops are enough. The use of these essential oils differs depending on the type of plant the oil is extracted from. One of the key questions one can ask is why have experts gone to such an extent to find treatment for stress? The answer is a simple one. In these modern times, stress has become a major problem. With the toughening economy and faster lifestyle, many people are finding it hard to cope. The failure to meet the daily expectations of a modern life and the pressure associated with striving to thrive in the busy world increasingly makes people prone to stress.

The normal person is not the only one that is subject to stress. People who work in the military and other related professions are prone to high-stress levels. The high levels of stress are pushing people to see therapists to help them cope with stress, and as such stress has become a medical problem. It is because of such reasons that experts have gone to such lengths to do intense research to find treatment for relieving stress. If stress is left unattended to, it can be very harmful to an individual. High levels of stress can affect the level of immunity in the body as well as predispose one to cardiovascular diseases (Rimmer, 2008).

One of the ways that oil from the aromatic plants can be used is by placing it in diffusers that allow it to slowly be released into the air. Whereas this may seem as a new way of dealing with stress, aromatherapy dates back to the ancient ages when Egyptians used it to improve their wellbeing through massage and healing (Buckle, 2003). Nowadays, one of the primary uses of aromatherapy is to manage stress levels.

Other than the use of diffusers, aromatherapy can be applied through inhalation and topical applications. In other cases such as in the healing of congestion and infections, the oils can be administered orally, rectally or even virginally. Although there can be aromatic oils that can be synthetically produced, experts choose to use the natural ones because the synthetic ones do not offer the same benefits. In fact, the synthetic oils have chemicals that may have irritation as a side effect (Alexander, 2001).

Aromatherapy also works with massage. As one of the primary stress relieving methodologies that have been used for centuries, massage works well with aromatherapy because it highly relies on the use of oils to rub body tissues to relaxation. Massage therapists can now use essential oils that are more inclined to soothing and distressing more than the normal oils. In case the massage therapist does not have some essential oils, one can go with their own essential oil to the parlor.

How Aromatherapy Works

First of all, aromatherapy is a very organic process that substitutes the use of manufactured pharmaceutical products for natural ingredients. By inhaling the oils from a reasonable distance, the elements in the oils reach the brain that reacts by slowing down, thus creating a relaxing effect. The oil can be applied to the body whereby it penetrates the skin through the hair follicles as well as the sweat glands. Then they are absorbed into the body fluids where they kill bacteria and stimulate the body immune system. Aromatherapy oil can be inhaled and the molecules absorbed into the body via nasal passage, the olfactory membrane, to the sinuses, then to trachea and finally reach the lungs.

Effects of stress on the body

Buckle (2015), defines stress as any change that makes the body adjust and react in a certain manner to the change. The body can react to these changes in various ways ranging from mental, physical to emotional responses. Stress can be of two forms: negative, also known as distress and positive which is also referred to as eustress. Positive stress can be from an example such getting a new job or being promoted. Negative stress is experienced when one is subjected to constant challenges without getting a relief in between. Such kind of straining makes one overworked and the body builds tension that needs to be released.

When distress mounts to high levels, one can start experiencing such symptoms as headaches, indigestion, insomnia or pain in the chest. People that have such conditions such as coronary diseases have a bigger problem as distress can aggravate their condition. Another danger of stress is when it is dealt with using inappropriate means such as smoking or drinking. Those that choose to use this method subject themselves to other harmful effects to their bodies such as cancer and alcohol-related accidents. Instead of such substances helping the body relax, the body ends up being in more stress. In fact, according to statistics, about 43% of adults experience ailments that are stress related. According to reports, stress is such a huge problem that costs the United States more than 300 billion dollars annually (Buckle, 2015).

Whereas it is nearly impossible to avoid moments that can subject one to stress, it is possible for one to choose to deal with the negative emotions that surround a situation. When stress goes to unmanaged levels, it can tamper with one's blood sugar levels thus making one hungry. This ultimately makes one be sensitive to insulin.

Cannard (2004) says that some other effects of stress are hard to detect. One may be lacking sleep or experiencing headaches that they may easily attribute to illnesses. Stress has been found to be a cause of such problems to many people. On another level, one may have reduced productivity due to their inability to focus and concentrate. One may also experience a reduced sex drive and muscle tension. When it comes to women, high levels of stress can have tamper with their menstrual cycle to have early or delayed periods.

The other effect of stress falls on the behavior of a person. One may be easily irritable, restless or have very low levels of motivation for work. It is quite easy for one to notice someone that is stressed because of the way they talk or relate to people or their work. Commonly, angry outbursts or withdrawal are common symptoms. The main challenge is in identifying oneself when under stress. Sometimes stress can lead to depression that drains one of their productivity. A depressed individual may seem to be sad most of the time (Rimmer, 2008).

The other effect of stress is on the immune system. In the short term, stress causes the immune system to be stronger. This makes the body heal wounds and kill infections. However, over a prolonged duration, the chemical cortisol negatively affects the immunity. It affects the body's ability to produce histamine and the body's general ability to respond to foreign infections. When one is under high stress, it is easy for them to contract such common illnesses such as influenza and common flue. This effect can also tamper with how long one takes to recover from illnesses already contracted.

One of the challenges that aromatherapy has faced as an alternative method of curing stress is that there is not sufficient scientific research that has been done to verify its effectiveness. As such, the use of these methodologies has not been yet fully embraced by many physicians and insurance companies (Morris, 2007).

One study was conducted by Sandra, Tara, Michelle, Carrie, & Eva (n.d). to test the effectiveness of the aromatic oils in the recovery of cardiac surgery patients. The study grouped the patients into randomly according to the type of oils they were using and whether or not they received massage therapy. The research did not find differences in the time taken for the patients to recover, but instead found that there were some key physiological differences among the various groups. Those patients that received the alternative treatment displayed more improvement physiologically as opposed to those that did not. The research also showed that the patients that were in the ICU that received aromatherapy using lavender had lower levels of anxiety and were in a better mood than those that did not undergo the therapy.

The study was undertaken using lavender as the main oil. This specifically has a reputation for having strong psychological effects in relieving stress and its effects such as irritability and panic. The study was aimed at finding out whether lavender can have psychological and physiological impacts on patients to remove acute stress and improve performance.

The conclusion of the study stated that whereas aromatherapy is an effective method of lowering stress and anxiety levels in patients, it is not highly effective in acute mental stress. The researchers also concluded that the application of aromatherapy was not found to be effective when applied to those undertaking math problems for a duration of 12 minutes. The findings indicated that aromatherapy had neither psychological nor physiological impact the subjects. The overall results concluded that when it comes to mental tasks, aromatherapy may not be effective in the short term but rather work well over the long term. The researchers also concluded that studies have not fully explored the effect of aromatherapy on acute stress levels.

Aromatherapy and mental health

Owing that over 60 % of total visits to doctors are stress related, many human trials have been conducted to see how much effective the practice is. It has been found that there are positive emotional effects. The potential of the practice is large as it can be used to deliver mental services to those that are highly stressed. If has been found that when some oils are inhaled, they can have significant impacts on alertness levels and anxiety. The oils further have been reported to have great impacts on some of the physical parameters of the nervous system. This causes relaxation. One interesting finding is that the use of the oil chamomile oil was found to induce stress levels in rats but serves as a mood booster in humans (Davidson, 2002).

The use of lavender has been found to have a positive impact on patients suffering from dementia especially the reduction of dementia. The same effects have been felt from the use of Melissa. It is not a wonder that some physicians in dementia care units have embraced the use of aromatherapy. The therapy has also been found to be very helpful in dealing with patients suffering from attention deficit-hyperactivity disorder. It has also been found to have a calming effect on those that have learning disorders by calming them (Balch, Stengler, & Young-Balch, 2011).

Modern research

The oils used in aromatherapy are volatile. The molecule contained in the substances then escape easily into the air. After breathing the molecules in, they go into the lungs and then flow into the blood stream. On reaching the brain, the molecules affect one's emotions, learning and memory amongst other brain functions. According to findings by Professor Hanns Hatt from Germany, the molecules from the aromatic oils act on the nerve cell receptors located in the brain. The other effect of the molecules is on the GABA neurotransmitter whose effect they increase (Buckle, 2015).

More research findings from Akio Nakamura say that some scents can change the gene activity and chemistry of the blood in such a way that they lower stress levels. The scientist together with others carried out an experiment on rats to determine whether the fragrances had any impact on the gene activity and blood chemistry. They examined two groups of rats that were under stress. One group was subjected to the fragrance linalool whereas the other was not. The findings showed that the rats that were exposed to linalool had a lower amount of two types of white blood cells to levels that were almost normal. The other rats had high levels of white blood cells due to the high levels of stress they were subjected to. The findings also indicated that linalool reduced the level of more than 100 genes that are normally high in times of stress. These findings were very important in identifying the types of fragrances that can be used to reduce stress levels in people.

The practice is also thought to work through the stimulation of receptors in the nose which send a message to the limbic system, which is the brain part that controls emotions. The oils can also enter the body through the skins by the rubbing of lotion, massage oils, and baths. The oils then move from the skin layers into the target muscles. Whereas most of the oils are stress relievers, there are others that are analgesic. These serve to relieve pain from muscles. Others are anti-anxiety, antibacterial, sedating, and anti-inflammatory (Bauer & Cutshall, n.d.).

Evidence of effectiveness

According to research by Professor Hanns Hatt, there were two fragrances that they found that had the same impact as the common drugs for calming people and inducing sleep. The fragrances were found to not only sooth people but also to promote sleep among the subjects. One of the strongest fragrances was jasmine. The two best fragrances were found to have an increase on the GABA neurotransmitter up to five times, thus serving just as well as the drugs. Further research by scientists from the Mia e University in Japan indicated an improvement on the levels of depression of patients that inhaled the citrus fragrance. The researchers said that the amount of anti-depressants that was required to treat the depression was reduced as a result of using the fragrance. The fragrance treatment was effective at lowering the levels of the neuroendocrine hormone (Buckle, 2015).

In another research in the US, a mixture of the essential oils lavender and rose were used to prevent postnatal depression. The women were required to use the fragrance for 15 minutes two times a week for a month. The research did not show any negative effects of the fragrance. In Australia, another research was conducted and found that among the 86 nurses that received aromatherapy massage and music therapy experienced lower stress levels than those that did not. The nurses worked in the accident and injuries department (Hinsdale, 2007).

Side effects and complications of aromatherapy

According to Doctor Brent A. Bauer, most of the essential oils have no side effects if used as directed by the doctor. However, other oils such as the tee tree, wormwood and tansy are poisonous and should strictly never be taken orally. Another possible associated effect of the use of the oils is fatigue and headaches. If one inhales too much of the oil, they can experience such effects. Another precaution that one should take is to realize how much concentrated and potent the oils are. They should be diluted before being used on the skin.

Other than the oils themselves, some people may react differently to the medication. One may have a negative reaction to one oil but not another. Before using the alternative oil, one should do a little test on their skins. This helps one to determine that they do not have an allergic reaction to the oil before applying it to the larger parts of the body. One should apply the oil to a small part of the body, usually the elbow and wait for 24 hours before determining whether they should proceed to use it in entirety. Among the effects to look out for are redness on the skin, sensations and sensitivity on exposure to the sun (Clarke, 2008).

Caution

Before a patient purchases and starts using a specific product, they should consult with their doctor. This will help the patient get the right guidance to avoid any possible allergic reaction or collision with some other medicine. Those for instance that are undergoing chemotherapy should undergo treatment to ensure that no reactions take place. Another case of patients are those that have high blood pressure. They should keep off fragrances that are made from rosemary and thyme. Those that suffer from diabetes should keep off the angelica oils. The last special group is pregnant women. Due to the many hormonal changes, such women should avoid using peppermint and rosemary (Clarke, 2008).

Conclusion

As discussed above, it is clear that aromatherapy is one of the alternative forms of treatment that is proving to be beneficial to many patients. The number of people affected by stress is very high. Aromatherapy has proven to be a medical field that can be further explored to build products that can help people deal with their day to day stress. One authorized by their doctor, one can identify the right fragrance for their soap, massage oil or candles. The work that has been done in coming up with the fragrances has proven to be very beneficial. With the advancement of technology, more fragrances can be found and newer products and forms of therapy developed to help soothe the many patients that are experiencing stress. The research indicates that not much has been done when it comes to acute stress. With the current technology and resources, more research is underway and researchers are confident to find ways of improving the lives of the many suffering patients.

References

Alexander, M. (2001). Aromatherapy & immunity: How the use of essential oils aid immune potentiality Part 2 mood-immune correlations, stress and susceptibility to illness and how essential oil odorants raise this threshold. *International Journal of Aromatherapy, 11*(3), 152-156. doi:10.1016/s0962-4562(01)80051-5

Balch, J. F., Stengler, M., & Young-Balch, R. (2011). *Prescription for natural cures: A self-care guide for treating health problems with natural remedies including diet, nutrition, supplements, and other holistic methods.* Hoboken: Wiley.

Bauer, B. A., & Cutshall, S. (n.d.). Aromatherapy. *The SAGE Encyclopedia of Theory in Counseling and Psychotherapy.* doi:10.4135/9781483346502.n27

Buckle, J. (2003). Clinical Use of Aromatherapy. *Clinical Aromatherapy,* 159-161. doi:10.1016/b978-044307236-9.50015-1

Buckle, J. (2015). Stress and Well-Being. *Clinical Aromatherapy,* 223-237. doi:10.1016/b978-0-7020-5440-2.00011-5

Cannard, G. (2004). The effect of aromatherapy in promoting relaxation and stress reduction in a general hospital. *Complementary Therapies in Nursing and Midwifery, 2*(2), 38-40. doi:10.1016/s1353-6117(96)80062-x

Clarke, S. (2008). Handling, safety and practical applications for use of essential oils. *Essential Chemistry for Aromatherapy,* 231-264. doi:10.1016/b978-0-443-10403-9.00008-x

Dasgupta, A., & Klein, K. (n.d.). *Antioxidants in food, vitamins and supplements: Prevention and treatment of disease.*

Davidson, J. (2002). Aromatherapy & work-related stress. *International Journal of Aromatherapy, 12*(3), 145-151. doi:10.1016/s0962-4562(02)00074-7

Hinsdale, R. (2007). *The use of aromatherapy, yoga, and foot massage as break-time stress reduction interventions for nurses.* Independence, MO: Graceland University.

Morris, N. (2007). Anxiety reduction by aromatherapy: Anxiolytic effects of inhalation of geranium and rosemary. *International Journal of Aromatherapy,*

Rimmer, L. (2008). The Clinical Use of Aromatherapy in the Reduction of Stress. *Home Healthcare Nurse: The Journal for the Home Care and Hospice Professional,*

Sandra, S.-E., Tara, F., Michelle, P., Carrie, B., & Eva, S (n.d). *STRESS MANAGEMENT:AROMATHERAPY AS AN ALTERNATIVE.* Pseudoscience and Psychotherapy.